Advance Praise for *Yoga for Pregnancy*

In *Yoga for Pregnancy*, Judith Lasater draws upon her experiences as a mother of three children, and her love of yoga practice and teaching. Her yoga program and "Mantras for Mom and Baby" will help pregnant women and new moms access the relief, relaxation, self-awareness, strength, and courage needed for motherhood.

—Regina Brunig, R.N.; labor and delivery nurse, and yoga teacher

Judith Lasater is a masterful yoga teacher who embodies the feminine. In this book, she brings together her vast knowledge, deep wisdom, and experience as a mother for the benefit of women and their babies. A pre- and postnatal yoga classic is born!

—Shiva Rea, yogini; featured in *Yoga Journal's Prenatal Yoga* and *Yoga Journal's Postnatal Yoga* (videos).

Judith Lasater is one of our country's master yoga teachers. Her primer is a much-needed addition to the books that truly help women prepare their bodies, minds, and spirits for the potentially transformative journey of birthing and mothering. And transformation is what it's is all about, isn't it!

—Suzanne Arms, author of *Immaculate Deception*

YOGA FOR PREGNANCY

Relax and Renew: Restful Yoga for Stressful Times (Rodmell Press, 1995)

Living Your Yoga: Finding the Spiritual in Everyday Life (Rodmell Press, 2000)

30 Essential Yoga Poses: For Beginning Students and Their Teachers (Rodmell Press, 2003)

Also by Judith Lasater, Ph.D., P.T.

rodmell press

YOGA SHORTS

YOGA

FOR PREGNANCY

WHAT EVERY MOM-TO-BE NEEDS TO KNOW

▼   ▼   ▼   ▼   ▼   ▼   ▼   ▼

Judith Lasater, Ph.D., P.T.

RODMELL PRESS   BERKELEY, CALIFORNIA, 2004

To my children:
Miles, Kam, and Elizabeth

▼　▼　▼　▼　▼　▼　▼　▼

Yoga for Pregnancy: What Every Mom-to-Be Needs to Know, copyright © 2004 by Judith Lasater, Ph.D., P.T. Photographs by Elise Browning Miller.

Rodmell Press Yoga Shorts

An earlier version of parts of this work appeared as an article in *Yoga Journal,* January–February 1994.

Library of Congress Cataloging-in-Publication Data

Lasater, Judith.
 Yoga for pregnancy : what every mom-to-be needs to
know / Judith Lasater.— 1st ed.
   p. cm. — (Rodmell Press yoga shorts)
 ISBN 1-930485-05-0 (paperback : alk. paper)
 1. Yoga. 2. Exercise for pregnant women. I. Title. II. Series.
 RG558.7.L373 2004
 618.2'44—dc22

                          2003026822

Printed in the United States of America
First Edition
ISBN 1-930485-05-0
10 09 08 07 06 05 04 1 2 3 4 5 6 7 8 9 10

Editor: Linda Cogozzo   Cover and Text Designer: Gopa & Ted2, Inc.

Copy Editor: Katherine L. Kaiser   Author Photographer: Elizabeth Lasater

Indexer: Ty Koontz   Cover and Interior Photographer:
Lithographer: Phoenix Color Corp.   Elise Browning Miller, www.embyoga.com

Text set in Dante

Contents

▼ ▼ ▼ ▼ ▼ ▼ ▼ ▼

Part Three

Acknowledgments

▼ ▼ ▼ ▼ ▼ ▼ ▼ ▼ ▼

IT IS WITH A FULL HEART that I acknowledge the extraordinary learning experience of being pregnant with my three children: Miles, Kam, and Elizabeth.

Thanks, too, to my husband, Ike, who not only lovingly contributed to their conception, but also stood by me during my pregnancies and labors.

I acknowledge my friends Toni Montez and Geri Herbert for their loving presence and hand-holding during my labors with Kam and Elizabeth.

Thanks to my friend Elise Browning Miller, yoga teacher and photographer, who shot the yoga photographs with good humor and skill, and to my daughter, Elizabeth, for her photograph of me. I appreciate yoga teacher Lisa Brill Robinson, who modeled for the "Yoga for Pregnancy, Labor, and Delivery" sequence, as well as yoga teacher Ruth Owen, who is pictured in the "Practicing Yoga After the Baby Arrives" sequence.

Namaste to Suzanne Arms, Regina Brunig, R.N., and Shiva Rea for their generous and heartfelt contributions to this work.

I am grateful each day to my first yoga teachers, Sally and David Ellsberry, and to B. K. S. Iyengar and his children, Geeta Iyengar and Prashant Iyengar.

My gratitude goes to my publishers, Donald Moyer and Linda Cogozzo, at Rodmell Press, as well as their team: copy editor Katherine L. Kaiser, indexer Ty Koontz, and designers Gopa and Veetam, at Gopa & Ted2, Inc.

Most of all, I thank my students—present and past—who have given me the gift of allowing me to teach them what is in my heart.

▼ ▼ ▼ ▼ ▼ ▼ ▼ ▼ ▼

Part One

Practicing Yoga for Pregnancy, Labor, and Delivery

▼ ▼ ▼ ▼ ▼ ▼ ▼ ▼ ▼ ▼ ▼ ▼ ▼ ▼ ▼ ▼ ▼ ▼ ▼ ▼

A FTER GOING THROUGH pregnancy, labor, and delivery with my three children, I can testify wholeheartedly to the tremendous value of a yoga practice for each of these three phases of becoming a mother. Conversely, I learned many things from my pregnancies that have helped me to practice yoga in a more committed and compassionate way.

Pregnancy taught me to accept each day as a new experience. When I was pregnant, I couldn't predict how my body would feel on any particular day, just as I can never predict how my yoga practice will go. Because of my yoga training, I was able to be more accepting of what was happening in my body, even as I marveled at the profound changes that were occurring.

Before I was pregnant, practicing unusual and sometimes demanding yoga poses (asana) taught me that I could trust my body. I had discovered that I could depend upon, as well as enjoy, my body as it stretched and let go into strange new positions. This sense of acceptance helped me to trust the process of pregnancy, to trust that my body would, miraculously and yet mundanely, grow a baby.

Labor, on the other hand, taught me more concentration than I had previously imagined possible! I continually used my yoga training to remember to connect my breathing with the uterine contractions during the hours required to give birth. Many times I reminded myself that each contraction was simply a difficult yoga pose, and that breathing, relaxation, and persistence would get me through it. Finally, the actual birth of our children gave me a greater understanding of the joy of life and a recommitment to opening my heart to the present moment, even if that moment was difficult or demanding. With each birth, my soul felt wiped clean for those few hours while I focused on the intensity of the moment. Without my yoga training, I'm not sure that I would have embraced the intensity so wholeheartedly or learned so much about myself. After these experiences, I know that practicing yoga is the perfect preparation for pregnancy, labor, and delivery.

How can a regular yoga class or a personal yoga practice specifically aid you as a pregnant woman? The most important way is by increasing your awareness of your mind and body. Moving the body into the various postures and sitting still in meditation involve observing the body, breath, and mind in action—as well as in interaction with one another. You learn to observe the tightness in your muscles, the restrictions of your breath, and the constant flow of your thoughts. Thus a yoga practice teaches you a new habit: the habit of clear self-perception, even during difficult moments. This habit of self-awareness is exactly what pregnancy, labor, delivery, and motherhood demand if these are to be healthy, rich, and fulfilling experiences. Living with clearer perception helps you to make conscious choices about health that will positively affect your body and your baby.

Practicing yoga helps you as a pregnant woman—whether you are an advanced practitioner or novice—in three other specific ways. The first benefit is physiological: yoga allows you especially to cultivate the art of relaxation. Relaxation is well documented as beneficial for health; it is especially salutary for the pregnant woman.

Fatigue is common during pregnancy, both because of the extra weight that is being carried and because of various hormonal changes that occur, especially in the first few months. I remember actually falling asleep at an important dinner during the first trimester of a pregnancy; I just got up from the table, found a bedroom, and went to sleep on the first bed that I saw. I couldn't help myself! This type of experience is more common earlier in pregnancy; fatigue from carrying extra weight occurs later in pregnancy. I used to dare my husband to strap a hefty backpack across his abdomen and carry it all day, even during sleep. (He politely declined.)

Yogic relaxation techniques can alleviate fatigue before it becomes incapacitating. Specific poses to enhance relaxation will be presented later, along with poses to help with some of the other common physiological trials of pregnancy. Besides fatigue, these common experiences include lower back pain, nausea and indigestion, swelling, and leg cramps.

The second major boon that the practice of yoga offers you as a pregnant woman is a balanced mental state. Yoga teaches that wholeness is experienced through a balance of focus (*abhyasa*) and surrender (*vairagya*). Without focus, a yoga pose has neither integrity nor stability; without surrender, it has neither heart and nor flow. In learning to balance focus and surrender, you become able to respond flexibly to the demands of the moment.

Labor exemplifies the need for this balance. During a contraction, your attention is naturally drawn inward strongly. The pain can be intense, but if you are able to stay focused on the sensations, breathing into them rather than running away from them, then you won't be overwhelmed: you will, like a surfer, ride the waves of pain, rather than drowning in them. Thus you will avoid or reduce the necessity for pain-relieving drugs during labor.

The use of drugs during labor can have deleterious effects on the baby, who is struggling so hard to be born. An unmedicated mother means an unmedicated baby, which most midwives and doctors will admit is almost always preferable. So the ability to focus during the difficulty of a labor contraction is as desirable as it is challenging. Learn to focus during the months of pregnancy, and you will carry this skill into labor.

But what happens between the contractions is equally important. The pause between contractions is the ideal opportunity for relaxation, Nature's way of providing a "time out" for the laboring woman. I can remember vividly how thankful I was for this little rest. If you have trained yourself to relax during the months of pregnancy, then you will find it easier to relax from the unremitting energy of the labor contraction when you have the chance, thus conserving your energy for the hard work ahead.

Finally, the practice of yoga offers the woman making the transition into motherhood a psychological advantage. There is nothing more demanding than the raising of a small child. Children don't understand that their parents sleep later than usual on Sunday, or that they may not want to play with them at 2:00 A.M. Most of all, children don't understand that their needs may be inconvenient, their crying unnerving, and their individual rhythms far from universal.

Because these demands are so fatiguing, both physically and emotionally, it's crucial for a mother to keep a strong sense of self. This means that you must have some time and space set aside just for you, time that is not spent mothering or partnering or working. Developing a yoga practice during pregnancy is an excellent way to start the habit of spending time *by yourself* and *for yourself.* Even 30 minutes of practice can change your mood and your outlook, as well as improve your health. When the demands of child rearing are at a fever pitch, it's comforting to know that you will have a period of time in which your attention will be on your own needs, not those of other people.

Practice

I have designed a sequence of yoga poses and other movements that can be practiced by students of all levels. (The Sanskrit name is given for each asana.) Please check with your health care professional before attempting them, with the possible exception of the Side-Lying Relaxation Pose (Figure 1), especially if there are any complications with your pregnancy. Remember to pay attention to your comfort at all times, and if these poses feel wrong or inappropriate for any reason, simply stop practicing. If possible, consult a trained yoga teacher and follow her advice as well.

You may find it beneficial to practice these poses and movements in the morning and again at night. Some women find that they like to spread them out through the day as their schedules permit. In any event, it's probably impossible to practice the Side-Lying Relaxation Pose too much!

Side-Lying Relaxation Pose

▼ ▼ ▼ ▼ ▼ ▼ ▼   ALLEVIATES FATIGUE

Props

• a carpeted floor • 1 nonskid mat • 1 wall
• 2 blankets • 2 bolsters • 3 pillows • 2 bath towels

Alternative Prop • a bed

Prop Note

Props can be used interchangeably. If you have more pillows, then you will need fewer blankets and vice versa.

The most important pose for pregnant women to practice every day is Side-Lying Relaxation Pose (Figure 1). It is a variation of the classic Corpse Pose (Savasana), or what I call Basic Relaxation Pose, which is practiced in a supine position. However, I do not recommend lying on your back during the last two trimesters of pregnancy, because it can cause the weight of the uterus to compress the vena cava, the major vein that returns the blood from the lower body to the heart.

Side-Lying Relaxation Pose is the magic elixir for pregnancy, labor, and the postpartum period. It can alleviate feelings of general fatigue, and is a good position for labor. I also found it to be a relaxing nursing position. When I nursed while lying on my side, I could use that time to feed and interact with the baby. Side-Lying Relaxation Pose also eased the tiredness I felt from late-night feedings.

Spread your nonskid mat on a carpeted floor and near a wall. Position a bolster so that when you lie down, the bolster is wedged between you and the wall and presses against your back. You will find the light pressure of the bolster to be both reassuring and relaxing. Have your other props close at hand.

Lie down on your side. Bend your knees and place a folded blanket or pillow between them, as well as some support, such as a folded bath towel, between your ankles. Take care not to position the top knee in front of the bottom knee in a way that torques the lower back. If you must move your leg forward to be comfortable, then be certain that the top knee is well supported and the lower back is not strained. Drape a blanket over your legs, which you will pull up once you have positioned the props for your head and arms.

FIGURE 1
SIDE-LYING RELAXATION POSE

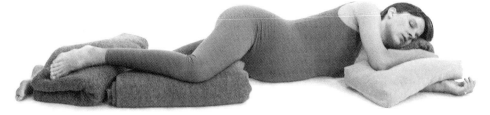

Place a folded blanket or pillow under your head and neck. Drape your upper arm over another bolster or pillow, or place a pillow between your arms. If you prefer to prop up your arms with the pillow, then place some support, such as a folded bath towel, under the bottom forearm.

Take a few moments to observe your posture. Make sure that your body is softly curved and that you feel completely supported by the props. You should feel as though you could fall asleep in this position. If you experience any discomfort in the shoulder that is resting on the floor, try practicing on your bed. Then learn to practice on the floor. It is a wonderful skill to be able to lie down anywhere and relax at will.

When you are comfortably positioned, close your eyes and pay particular attention to relaxing the jaw, the belly, the hands, and the breath. Allow yourself to receive the support of the floor.

Paradoxically, one of the best ways to relax is simply to become aware of your tension. Whenever you become completely aware of your tension, it immediately begins to ebb. Take slow and long breaths at first, gradually letting your breathing assume a natural rhythm. Spend some of this quiet, relaxing time in unspoken communication with your unborn child. This is a time when you could practice a "Mantra for Mom and Baby," which I describe in Part Three (see page 51). Even if you don't practice with a mantra, send your child feelings of welcoming and love.

Let the sounds around you simply drift past: no need to interact with them. Feel the innate perfection of this moment of relaxation. Remain in Side-Lying Relaxation Pose for 20 to 30 minutes. When you are ready to come out of the pose, slowly open your eyes. Gradually sit up, taking care to use your arms to help yourself to a sitting position. Using your arms in this way will help to protect your lower back and abdomen from strain.

After you have come out of the pose, you may feel a little spacey. Give yourself some time before you try to drive or cope with other complicated tasks. Practice Side-Lying Relaxation Pose on alternating sides of the body each day, the right side one day and the left side the following day, unless you very strongly prefer one side. I cannot emphasize enough how important it is to practice this pose every day. Remember this pose for the most intense part of labor.

Cat–Cow Stretch

▼ ▼ ▼ ▼ ▼ LESSENS LOWER
BACK PAIN

Props

• a carpeted floor • 1 nonskid mat

Most pregnant women experience some degree of lower back pain during pregnancy, either occasionally or for more extended periods. No wonder, considering the biomechanics of the pregnant body. Greatly increased weight is concentrated just opposite the lower back, one of the weaker areas of the spine. At the same time, the abdominal muscles, which usually add support to the

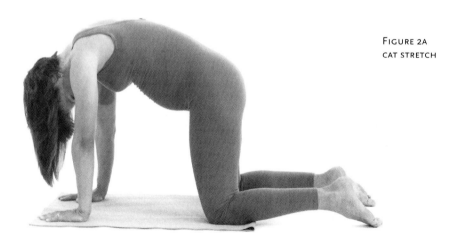

FIGURE 2A
CAT STRETCH

trunk, are greatly stretched, thus compromising their support function. By the end of pregnancy, the size of the belly may make everyday tasks, such as washing dishes, challenging: the pregnant woman may need to practically stand sideways to reach the sink of dishes over her belly. Such body mechanics put considerable strain on the muscles and ligaments of the lower back.

One of the best movements for the lower back is Cat–Cow Stretch (Figure 2A and Figure 2B). Place your nonskid mat on a carpeted floor. Kneel on your mat, placing the hands under the shoulders and the knees a little wider than the hips. Begin by turning your awareness to your breath. After several easy breaths, exhale and drop the head and the tailbone downward, rounding the belly slightly upward (Figure 2A). The spine is now in the shape of a cat's back. With an inhalation, immediately reverse the spinal position lifting the head and tailbone

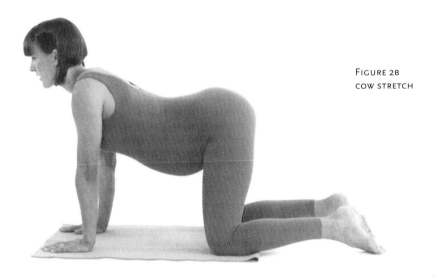

FIGURE 2B
COW STRETCH

and dropping the belly so that it resembles the back of a cow (Figure 2B). Repeat these movements ten to twenty times, coordinating them with the breath. Be careful not to force the spine downward: rather, gently press it into an even arch. Think of originating the movement from the front of the body, the belly.

Not only does Cat–Cow Stretch relieve the lower back, it also can help to relieve a cramp in the round ligament, which connects the uterus to the sacrum. This ligament is unique in the body because, like a muscle, it contains some contractile tissue. A pregnant women will occasionally get a cramp in the round ligament when the enlarged uterus shifts suddenly, for example, when she stands up quickly from lying down. This cramp manifests as a sharp, stabbing pain in the lower and outer quadrant of the abdomen, either on the right or on the left. The Cow–Cat Pose can help to alleviate this pain.

A word to seasoned practitioners: Do not underrate these movements. When I was pregnant for the first time, they were recommended to me, but I dismissed them as too simple, a waste of time. When I finally tried Cat–Cow Stretch, I found it not only effective for my lower back and round ligaments, but enjoyable as well. Try it before bed to reduce any residual tension in the lower back created by carrying the baby in your belly all day.

After you have repeated this pose with the breathing a few times, pause with the spine in a neutral position for a few moments and observe how you feel. Carefully stand up, or proceed with the next pose.

Reclining Heroine Pose

▼ ▼ ▼ ▼ ▼ ▼ RELIEVES NAUSEA
AND INDIGESTION

Props
- a carpeted floor • 1 nonskid mat
- 3 to 4 blankets • 1 bolster • 1 pillow

Possible Props
- 1 block, or 1 book, or 1 blanket

The most unpopular companions of many pregnancies are, no doubt, nausea and indigestion. Doctors will tell you that progesterone, the hormone that causes morning sickness, is the same one that helps to maintain a healthy pregnancy. This good news is not an unmixed blessing for the woman who feels as though she has the flu or a hangover for days, weeks, or even months at a time. Many alternative health care practitioners have theories about why pregnant women suffer from nausea or indigestion, generally attributing it to an imbalance in nutrition or energy. Morning sickness may be Nature's way of preventing the pregnant woman from ingesting poisonous substances. Whatever the cause, these symptoms are certainly unpleasant and can even be dangerous if the woman is unable to eat enough to provide for the growing baby.

A yoga pose that many expectant mothers use to combat nausea (as well as reduce indigestion, which can be caused by the pressure of the expanded uterus on the internal organs) is Reclining Heroine Pose (Supta Virasana, Figure 3A). In traditional yoga texts, this pose is translated as Hero Pose, but in light of the challenge presented by pregnancy, labor, and delivery, I have renamed it in the feminine, that is, Heroine Pose. On many mornings during my pregnancies, I practiced this pose before I even got out of bed.

Place your nonskid mat on a carpeted floor, and place the folded blankets on the mat and under a bolster. Kneel in front of the bolster, and sit down between your heels. If this position is uncomfortable, then place a block (or a book or a folded blanket) under your buttocks to eliminate knee pain. Make sure that your feet point straight back and do not splay at 90 degrees to the lower leg.

Lie back on the bolster, and place a pillow under your head. An important

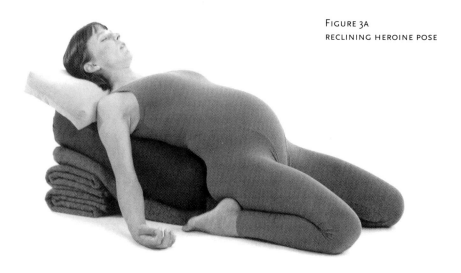

FIGURE 3A
RECLINING HEROINE POSE

detail is to support the lower back fully with the blankets so that there is no gap between the mat and the lumbar spine. Notice how, in Figure 3A, the model's back is held firmly by the bolster and blankets. Make sure that your torso is arranged so that the forehead is higher than the chin, the chin higher than the breastbone, and the breastbone higher than the pelvis. Common misalignments in this pose are to raise the head too high with the chin dropped and to place the body too flat on the floor. (See Figure 3B, which shows the *incorrect* way to practice.) Think of this pose as halfway between sitting and lying, as if you were reclining in a chaise longue.

The final position should be soothing and comfortable. Close your eyes and breathe slowly. In a good Reclining Heroine Pose, the ribs are slightly flared

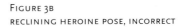

FIGURE 3B
RECLINING HEROINE POSE, INCORRECT

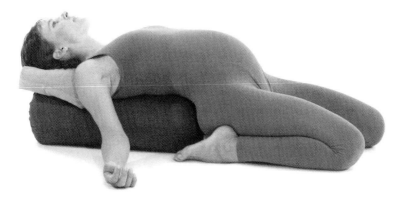

and lifted away from the stomach and liver. Remain in the pose for 3 to 10 minutes, depending on your level of experience. Be sure to use your arms to support yourself as you come up. Then place your hands in front of you on the floor, so that you're on all fours, and stand up slowly.

Many students find that this position is particularly helpful for nausea, but it can be used for simple indigestion as well. The knees should not hurt: if they do, raise the height under the buttocks. If this modification doesn't alleviate the discomfort, then seek out the aid of a trained yoga teacher.

Wall Stretch

Props

• 1 nonskid mat • 1 wall

Few things could be as unpleasant as being awakened from blissful slumber by the stabbing, squeezing pain of a cramp in the calf muscles. Once you've experienced this, as many pregnant women do, you will have a new respect for your own muscle strength. The calves, made up principally of the gastrocnemius and soleus muscles, are especially prone to nocturnal cramping. It's quite a shock to be sound asleep one minute and hopping around the bedroom screaming in pain the next.

What has occurred is that the muscles in the lower leg have contracted and refused to let go. One theory is that reduced circulation during sleep creates the cramp; another theory is that inadequate calcium in the bloodstream causes the muscle filaments to remain contracted. Whatever the cause, Wall Stretch (Figure 4A) is an effective solution.

Wall Stretch is both preventive and curative. I suggest that you practice this pose several times during the day, as well as make use of it to resolve a night cramp, should one occur.

Position your nonskid mat on a level surface, with the short end near a wall. Stand on the mat, facing the wall, with one foot back and one foot forward.

Raise your arms to shoulder level, and press your hands against the wall. Make sure that your back foot is 90 degrees to the wall and that the heel is not turned in at an angle. If you keep the foot straight, then the stretch will be more effective. Press the heel down and breathe normally. Keep your body upright and the shoulders back: don't lean forward toward the wall. Hold the pose for several minutes, feeling a strong but pleasant stretch in the lower portion of the back leg.

An interesting variation is to bend the back knee while keeping the heel on

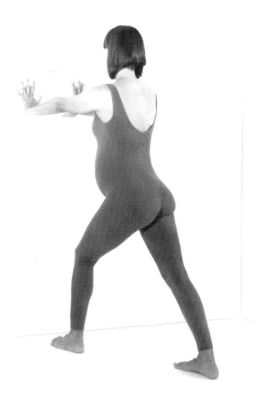

FIGURE 4A
WALL STRETCH

the floor (Figure 4B). This stretches the gastrocnemius muscles, instead of the soleus muscles. Some people find that one of these stretches is much stronger than the other. If this is true for you, then spend more time stretching the tighter area.

Whether you are practicing the main movement or its variation, after several minutes of stretching one lower leg, switch to the other. Make sure that you spend the same amount of time stretching the second leg as you spent on the first one. After you have finished stretching, take a few steps around the room, and feel the ease with which you walk. If you're awakened in the middle of the night with a cramp, remember this pose. It will help tremendously.

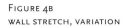
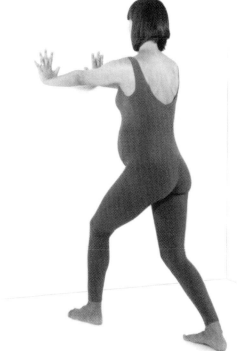

FIGURE 4B
WALL STRETCH, VARIATION

Bound-Angle Pose

▼ ▼ ▼ ▼ ▼ ▼   PREPARES YOU
FOR LABOR

Props

• 1 nonskid mat • a carpeted floor • 1 to 3 blankets

Although labor composes a short period of your life, it's obviously a significant
one. Bound-Angle Pose (Baddha Konasana, Figure 5A) is an excellent preparation for labor: it improves your ability to open your legs and allow for the

FIGURE 5A
BOUND-ANGLE POSE

FIGURE 5B
BOUND-ANGLE POSE, INCORRECT

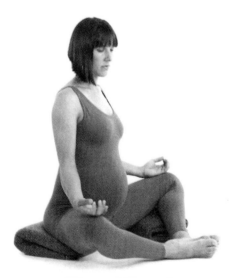

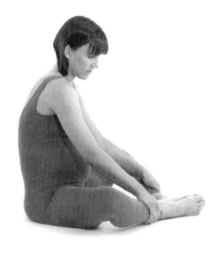

passage of the baby. If you're flexible in this region, then you will be able to maintain this open position with more relaxation for a longer period of time. Place your nonskid mat on a carpeted floor. Sit on the mat and place the soles of your feet together, letting the knees drop out to the sides. Breathe normally and quietly. Pay attention to the curve of the lower back. If the lower back is rounding out and the spine is sinking (Figure 5B, incorrect), then sit on the edge of one or two folded blankets, so that the lower back can assume a normal inward curve. Be careful to keep the spine curved inward to avoid straining the lower back. Place the arms in a comfortable position, either holding the feet or resting on the thighs. If you experience discomfort in one of the knees or inner thighs, or if one knee is much farther down than the other, then place a rolled blanket under that leg for support, as shown in Figure 5A.

Sit in this pose whenever you have the opportunity. Vary the pose by placing the feet slightly farther from or slightly closer to the body, thus stretching a different part of the hip joints and muscles. Stay in Bound-Angle Pose for several minutes. Incorporate this pose into your daily life, for example, while watching television or folding laundry.

To come out of the pose, place the arms around the outsides of the thighs, lift them up, and bring them together. This technique will lessen the possibility of stressing the ligaments around the pubic bone. Rest for a moment before getting up or proceeding to the next pose.

Side-Lying Inversion

▼ ▼ ▼ ▼ REDUCES SWELLING
IN THE LEGS

Props

- a carpeted floor • 1 nonskid mat
- 1 wall • 5 to 7 blankets • 2 bolsters
- 1 to 4 pillows • 2 bath towels

Prop Note

Props can be used interchangeably. If you have more pillows, then you will need fewer blankets and vice versa.

Many pregnant women complain of swelling in the legs and ankles, especially in the latter part of pregnancy and during hot weather. Excessive swelling can indicate serious problems with the maternal circulatory system and requires the prompt attention of a health care professional. But this simple inverted posture can help with the slight normal swelling that many experience.

Because the classic inverted poses of Headstand (Salamba Sirsasana) and Shoulderstand (Salamba Sarvangasana) are difficult, even contraindicated, for pregnant women, I recommend Side-Lying Inversion (Figure 6).

Spread your nonskid mat on a carpeted floor. Begin in Side-Lying Relaxation Pose (Figure 1) and prop yourself accordingly. Place your calves on a stack of folded blankets. In this position, the feet are approximately 6 inches above the level of the head. Prop the head and arms comfortably with folded blankets or with pillows.

Remain in this pose for 10 to 15 minutes. Let all the sounds around you simply drift past, without interacting with them. Feel the innate perfection of this moment of relaxation. As you lie there, take those moments to tune into your growing baby. In a way that feels appropriate to you, connect with your baby. Maybe you visualize your baby nestled inside you, sleeping. Maybe you imagine your baby snuggled asleep beside your body in the months after birth. Maybe you see your family with the addition of this new life. Whatever you imagine, let these precious moments be ones of welcoming and ease. Remember to breathe softly and easily.

To come out of the pose, carefully move your legs to the side and lie on a level surface for several minutes before using your arms to help yourself up to a sitting position.

FIGURE 6
SIDE-LYING INVERSION

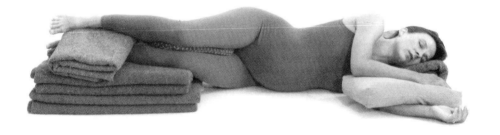

One of the paradoxes of pregnancy is that to the woman it seems to pass slowly, while to those around her it passes quickly. Labor, however, often seems to go slowly for all involved. Whatever your perceptions about the duration of pregnancy, labor, and delivery, yoga can help you to feel better throughout them and enjoy the processes as much as possible. Ideally, the habit of taking care of your body, which you've cultivated by practicing yoga, will extend past giving birth into the process of parenting. Conscious parenting is the ultimate yoga practice.

▼   ▼   ▼   ▼   ▼   ▼   ▼   ▼   ▼

Part Two

Practicing Yoga After the Baby Arrives

▼ ▼ ▼ ▼ ▼ ▼ ▼ ▼ ▼ ▼ ▼ ▼ ▼ ▼ ▼ ▼

I T IS NO OVERSTATEMENT to say that when you have a baby everything changes. One of these changes is your priorities: suddenly the small creature whom you hold in your arms is the center of your life and thoughts. What many women find is that they begin to lose interest in themselves. A certain amount of this is normal. However, choosing to care for yourself is the best way to make sure that your baby and family have the finest care. When you are a little more rested, refreshed, and centered, your child and family reap the benefits. And as your child grows, you will be modeling the importance of self-care, teaching him or her to pay attention to health and inner states.

Your yoga practice sustained you during your pregnancy; let it sustain you afterward. Try to work out a strategy with your partner, a friend, or a relative that includes a few minutes every day for you to get back on the mat. Once your life is beginning to settle into a routine—as much as it can with a newborn—you may wonder how you can get your body back to its prepregnancy shape and energy level.

To reduce fatigue, I recommend that you continue practicing Side-Lying Relaxation Pose (Figure 1). To increase energy, I suggest taking daily walks. Walking improves muscle strength and endurance, keeps the heart and respiratory system healthy, burns calories, and improves your mood. Put the baby into a baby carrier or stroller, and enjoy the fresh air.

To resume a yoga practice, try the poses given here. Use caution when beginning to practice postpartum. After birth, women experience a uterine blood flow, called the lochia, which can continue for up to six weeks. Do not practice any classical inversion poses until this flow has stopped. Other gentle poses are fine, but monitor the effect of your yoga practice on the lochia. If the flow increases or changes quality dramatically, then consult your health care professional and back off on the poses for a few days. Common sense will guide you.

Another note of caution concerns practicing sit-ups in the immediate postpartum period. Although sit-ups may seem to be the logical way to strengthen abdominal muscles postpartum, I do not recommend them. The muscles have been weakened by the increasing stretch that they have undergone for nine months, and sit-ups can strain them.

Remember that the abdominal muscles attach to the pubic bone, and the ligaments that hold the two halves of the pubic bone together have been loosened by hormonal changes. An active sit-up program practiced too soon postpartum can pull on the pubic bone, causing pelvic misalignment and sacroiliac pain. Get stronger first by walking and by performing the activities of daily living before you attempt sit-ups.

Practice

Three yoga poses that can be practiced as soon as you feel ready are Half-Dog Pose (Adho Mukha Svanasana, Figure 7), Warrior II Pose (Virabhadrasana II, Figure 8), and Seated-Twist Pose (Bharadvajasana, Figure 9). If you are an experienced yoga practitioner, then gradually add standing poses, forward bends and twists, simple backbends, and, finally, inversions. Your yoga practice will be even sweeter now that your time has more demands placed on it. But no matter how much you practice, the most important thing is to enjoy yourself and your baby.

Half-Dog Pose

▼ ▼ ▼ ▼ FOR FLEXIBILITY

Props

• 1 nonskid mat • 1 wall

Alternative Prop

• Edge of a kitchen sink

Half-Dog Pose (Adho Mukha Svanasana, Figure 7) can be practiced anywhere that there is a wall. Place your nonskid mat with the short end against a wall. Stand facing the wall and place your hands on it, so that they are shoulder-width apart and slightly lower than shoulder level. Keeping your breathing relaxed, slowly step back, sliding your hands down the wall until the torso and legs form a 90-degree angle. Firmly press away from the wall, so that the back lengthens and the shoulders drop.

Let the head drop down to stretch the back of the neck. Keep the knees straight and the feet directed straight ahead. Hold the pose for a few minutes, still keeping the breathing easy and natural. You will feel a stretch in the shoulders and perhaps in the backs of the legs. If you wish, exhale strongly and draw the abdomen toward the backbone, holding it in for just a moment. This will help to strengthen the abdominal muscles.

To come out of the pose, simply walk toward the wall while inhaling. Stand still for a moment and breathe deeply. If you feel any dizziness while coming up, then discontinue the practice of the pose for a few days before trying it again. Alternatively, you can practice Half-Dog Pose at the kitchen sink; your hands will fit perfectly over the edge of the sink.

Practice Half-Dog Pose several times during the day to alleviate any tension or fatigue in the upper back and shoulders that is created by carrying and nursing the baby. To prevent this tension in the first place, make sure that when you nurse, you use pillows to hold the baby up to the breast, so that you are not required to lean down toward the baby. Better yet, nurse your baby while practicing Side-Lying Relaxation Pose (Figure 1).

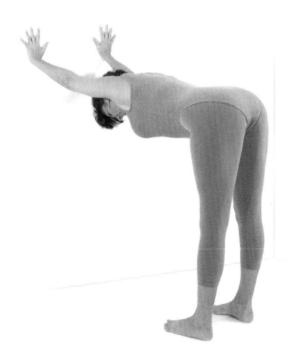

FIGURE 7
HALF-DOG POSE

Warrior II Pose

▼ ▼ ▼ ▼ ▼   FOR STRENGTH

Prop

- 1 nonskid mat

To practice Warrior II Pose (Virabhadrasana II, Figure 8), spread your nonskid mat on a level surface. Stand on the mat with your feet 4 to 4½ feet apart, turning the left foot in and the right foot out at 90 degrees. Check that the heel of

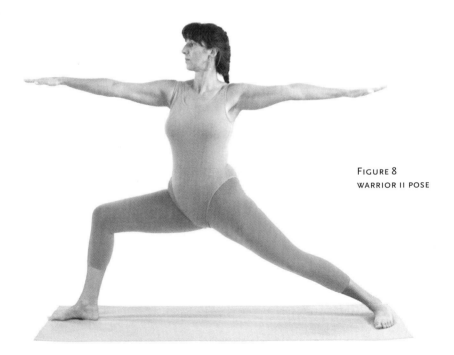

FIGURE 8
WARRIOR II POSE

the right foot is in a straight line with the middle of the arch of the back foot. Stretch the arms strongly out to the side, allowing your heart to lift up as you inhale. With an exhalation, gradually bend the right knee to a right angle, keeping the kneecap pointing over the little toe. The right thigh should be parallel with the floor. Keep the left knee straight. Turn the head to look over the right arm. Try to keep the torso facing forward, not twisted toward the right, and stretch back through the left arm.

Hold the pose for several breaths; before you tire, come out of the pose with an exhalation. Rest for a moment before practicing Warrior II Pose on the other side. This pose will strengthen the legs and abdomen; it will also increase endurance and confidence.

Seated-Twist Pose

▼ ▼ ▼ ▼ ▼ FOR ABDOMINAL
MUSCLE STRENGTH

Props
• 1 nonskid mat • 1 blanket • 1 wall

A gentle way to strengthen the abdomen is with Seated-Twist Pose (Bharadva-jasana, Figure 9), because twisting movements require the action of the abdominal muscles. Place your nonskid mat on a level surface. Sit with your right side about 6 inches from the wall, and fold your legs under to your left side. If your back rounds or the position feels strained, then place a folded blanket under just the right buttock to level the pelvis and help you to lift your spine. Your right shoulder should be near the wall, but not touching it.

Place the hands on the wall at shoulder height, making sure that the hands are spread apart so that the elbows are comfortably bent. Do not straighten the arms, because this action could strain the elbows. Inhale, and with the exhalation, gradually use the pressure of the right hand against the wall to help you turn toward it. The twist should begin low in the abdomen and spiral up the trunk. It is fine to feel a little more weight on the right buttock as you twist, but don't let the left buttock come completely off the floor.

With each exhalation, bring the abdomen in toward the spine for a moment and hold it firmly; this action will strengthen the abdominal muscles and put gentle pressure on the uterus. Then relax and breathe normally before trying this again. Stay in the pose for several breaths, twisting until your left shoulder moves near the wall. Come out of the pose with an exhalation. Practice the twist on the other side for the same number of breaths.

Never end your practice with a twist, because it leaves the spine in an uneven state. You can follow Seated-Twist Pose with Half-Dog Pose (Figure 7), with Side-Lying Relaxation Pose (Figure 1), or with both.

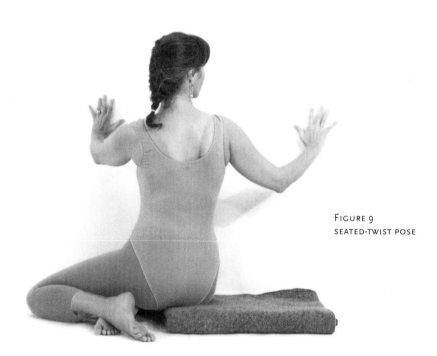

FIGURE 9
SEATED-TWIST POSE

Part Three

Mantras for Mom and Baby

▼ ▼ ▼ ▼ ▼ ▼ ▼ ▼ ▼ ▼ ▼ ▼

I N TWO OF MY BOOKS, *Living Your Yoga: Finding the Spiritual in Everyday Life* and *30 Essential Yoga Poses: For Beginning Students and Their Teachers,* I include, respectively, "Mantras for Daily Living" and "Mantras for Daily Practice." They reflect my experience that a sound or sentence that is repeated—in the yoga tradition, a mantra—can help to transform thoughts and consciousness. Pregnancy is a great time to use the power of the mind to create an environment of health and well-being for both you and your child.

Try these simple "Mantras for Mom and Baby" during your pregnancy and after the baby arrives. (Alternatively, you can compose your own mantras.) They can be helpful whenever you feel a little down or anxious, as well as when you want to celebrate the miracle of new life. You can say them either aloud or silently when you wake up, begin your yoga practice, step into the shower, come to a stoplight, relax, or drift off to sleep. Say them often to increase their power. The most important thing is to choose thoughts that enhance your life.

During Pregnancy

FIRST MONTH

I welcome life as it grows in my belly.

SECOND MONTH

Napping every day is vital to my well-being.

THIRD MONTH

Change is not just the way that it is: it is the *only* thing that is.

FOURTH MONTH

Letting go is the key to happiness.

FIFTH MONTH

When I rest, I am doing the most important thing
in the world right now.

SIXTH MONTH

New body, new hopes.

SEVENTH MONTH

Roundness is the ultimate feminine shape.

EIGHTH MONTH

My labor, however it goes, is perfect for me.

NINTH MONTH

My baby and I are connected in love.

During the First Year

FIRST MONTH

I celebrate the wonder of my new baby.

SECOND MONTH

I will rest with every breath.

THIRD MONTH

I can do this.

FOURTH MONTH

It won't always be like this.

FIFTH MONTH

I can let go of worry.

SIXTH MONTH

Practicing just three yoga poses can change my day.
I will practice three poses today.

SEVENTH MONTH

Watching my breath can help me get through my day with less stress.

EIGHTH MONTH

I will play with my baby for 20 minutes and let go of my need
to accomplish anything else at the same time.

Ninth Month

I will take some time to nurture myself.

Tenth Month

I will do ten sit-ups, ten push-ups, and ten minutes
of singing in the shower to celebrate my baby's tenth month.

Eleventh Month

I will lie down with my feet up for 5 minutes.

Twelfth Month

I will celebrate my first year of mothering
by taking a nap two times per week.

Resources

▼ ▼ ▼ ▼ ▼ ▼ ▼ ▼ ▼ ▼

Yoga with Judith Lasater

Judith Lasater offers ongoing yoga classes, leads yoga vacations, lectures and teaches at yoga conferences, and gives workshops and seminars, including Relax and Renew Seminars® and Living Your Yoga Seminars®. All are open to interested individuals, yoga teachers, and health care professionals.

Visit www.judithlasater.com for more information.

Books

Lasater, Judith, Ph.D., P.T. *30 Essential Yoga Poses: For Beginning Students and Their Teachers.* Berkeley, Calif.: Rodmell Press, 2003. (800) 841–3123, www.rodmell press.com.

———. *Living Your Yoga: Finding the Spiritual in Everyday Life.* Berkeley, Calif.: Rodmell Press, 2000. (800) 841–3123, www.rodmellpress.com.

———. *Relax and Renew: Restful Yoga for Stressful Times.* Berkeley, Calif.: Rodmell Press, 1995. (800) 841–3123, www.rodmellpress.com.

Mantra Mats™

Inspire your yoga practice with Judith Lasater's Mantra Mats™. Each mat is silk-screened with a "Mantra for Daily Living," from her *Living Your Yoga*. Contact Hugger-Mugger Yoga Products at (800) 473–4888 or visit www.huggermug ger.com.

Other Recommended Resources

Book

Englund, Pam, C.N.M., M.A., and Rob Horowitz, Ph.D. *Birthing from Within: An Extra-Ordinary Guide to Childbirth Preparation*. Albuquerque, N.M.: Partera Press, 1998.

Video

Arms, Suzanne. *Giving Birth: Challenges and Choices*.
(877) 247-8446,
www.birthingthefuture.com.

Magazines

The following yoga periodicals have published articles by Judith Lasater:

Ascent
www.ascentmagazine.com

LA Yoga
www.layogapages.com

Yoga Chicago
www.yogachicago.com

Yoga International
www.yimag.org

Yoga Journal
www.yogajournal.com

Where to Find a Yoga Teacher Online

www.yogaalliance.com • www.yogajournal.com • www.yogaassoc.com

About the Author

▼ ▼ ▼ ▼ ▼ ▼ ▼ ▼ ▼ ▼

Judith Lasater has taught yoga since 1971. She holds a doctorate in East–West psychology and is a physical therapist. She is president of the California Yoga Teachers Association, and serves on the advisory boards of *Yoga Journal* and the Yoga Research and Education Center.

Her yoga training includes study with B. K. S. Iyengar in India and the United States. She teaches yoga classes and trains yoga teachers in kinesiology, yoga therapeutics, and the Yoga Sutra in the San Francisco Bay Area. She also gives workshops throughout the United States, and has taught in Canada, England, France, Indonesia, Japan, Mexico, Peru, and Russia.

She writes extensively on the therapeutic aspects of yoga. She is the author of *Relax and Renew: Restful Yoga for Stressful Times* (1995), which is the first book devoted exclusively to the supported yoga poses and breathing techniques that make up restorative yoga; *Living Your Yoga: Finding the Spiritual in Everyday Life* (2000); and *30 Essential Yoga Poses: For Beginning Students and Their Teachers* (2003), all published by Rodmell Press.

Her popular "Asana" column ran in *Yoga Journal* for thirteen years, and she continues to contribute articles on a variety of subjects. In addition, her writing has appeared in numerous magazines and books, including *Yoga Interna-*

tional, Natural Health, Sports Illustrated for Women, Prevention, Alternative Thera-pies, Numedx, International Journal of Yoga Therapy (formerly *The Journal of the International Association of Yoga Therapists*), *Complementary Therapies in Rehabil-itation* (Slack), *Living Yoga* (Jeremy P. Tarcher/Perigee), *American Yoga* (Grove Press), *The New Yoga for People Over 50* (Health Communications), and *Lilias, Yoga, and Your Life* (Macmillan).

Judith Lasater lives in the San Francisco Bay Area with her family.

Yoga with Judith Lasater

Judith Lasater offers ongoing yoga classes, leads yoga vacations, lectures and teaches at yoga conferences, and gives workshops and seminars, including Relax and Renew Seminars® and Living Your Yoga Seminars®. All are open to inter-ested individuals, yoga teachers, and health care professionals.

Visit www.judithlasater.com for more information.

From the Publisher

▼ ▼ ▼ ▼ ▼ ▼ ▼ ▼ ▼

RODMELL PRESS publishes books on yoga, Buddhism, and aikido. In the Bhaga-vadgita it is written, "Yoga is skill in action." It is our hope that our books will help individuals develop a more skillful practice—one that brings peace to their daily lives and to the Earth.

We thank all whose support, encouragement, and practical advice sustain us in our efforts. In particular, we are grateful to Reb Anderson, B. K. S. Iyengar, Wendy Palmer, and Yvonne Rand for their inspiration.

To request a catalog or be on our e-announcements list, contact us at:

(510) 841–3123 or (800) 841–3123

(510) 841–3191 (fax)

info@rodmellpress.com

www.rodmellpress.com

Index